The Perfect Cookbook for Kidney Disease Patients

More than 20 Delicious and Healthy
Recipes

By

Heston Brown

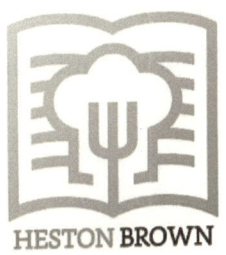

HESTON BROWN

Thank you so much for buying my book! I want to give you a special gift!

Receive a special gift as a thank you for buying my book. Now you will be able to benefit from free and discounted book offers that are sent directly to your inbox every week.

To subscribe simply fill in the box below with your details and start reaping the rewards! A new deal will arrive every day and reminders will be sent so you never miss out. Fill in the box below to subscribe and get started!

https://heston-brown.getresponsepages.com

Subscribe
to our
newsletter

Your Email

Table of Contents

Chapter I: Healthy Food Items for People with Kidney Disease

xxxxxxxxxxxxxxxxxxxxxxxxxxxxxxxx

There is a strong link between super foods, inflammation, and chronic disease because these elements can provide protection against fatty acid oxidation. It is a condition in which oxygen reacts with the fat in your blood and blood cells. Oxidation is a typical procedure to produce energy and control various chemical reactions in your body. Excessive oxidation of cholesterol and fat can create molecules called free radicals. These free radicals can damage your cell membranes, genes, and protein. Oxidative damage is directly linked to cancer, heart disease, Parkinson, Alzheimer and other chronic conditions. If you are suffering from chronic kidney disease, you should pay special attention to your diet. There are various things that are good for your health, but at the same time, a few things should be completely avoided:

(1) Green Cabbage

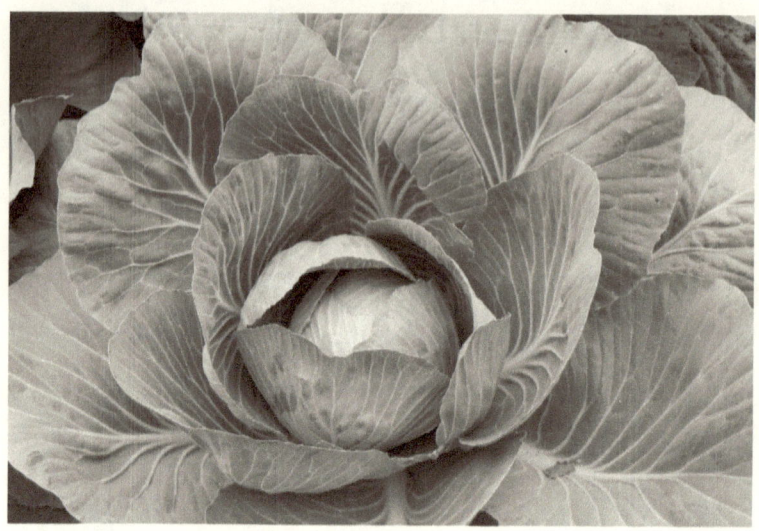

½ cup cabbage contains:

- Sixty milligrams Potassium
- Six milligram Sodium
- Nine-milligram phosphorus

Cabbage is a cruciferous vegetable that is packed with phytochemicals and useful chemical compounds. These compounds can break free radicals to avoid any damage in your body. Phytochemicals have the ability to fight cancer and improve cardiovascular health.

It is high in fiber, Vitamin K, and Vitamin C. It is a good source of folic acid and vitamin B6. Cabbage is a good source of folic acid and vitamin B6. It will be a good addition to your diet. You can eat raw cabbage or prepare cabbage soup, microwave it, steam or boil it. Add cheese and butter to enhance its taste and flavor.

(2) Garlic

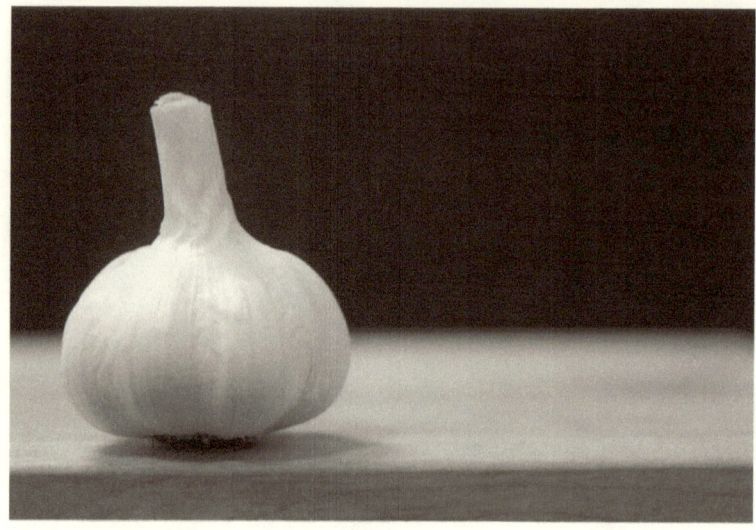

Only one clove of garlic has 12 milligrams potassium, 1-milligram sodium, and 4-milligram phosphorus. Garlic can be a good choice to avoid the formation of plaques in your teeth, reduce inflammation and cholesterol. Garlic powder will be an excellent substitute for garlic salt in a diet for dialysis patients.

(3) Red Bell Peppers

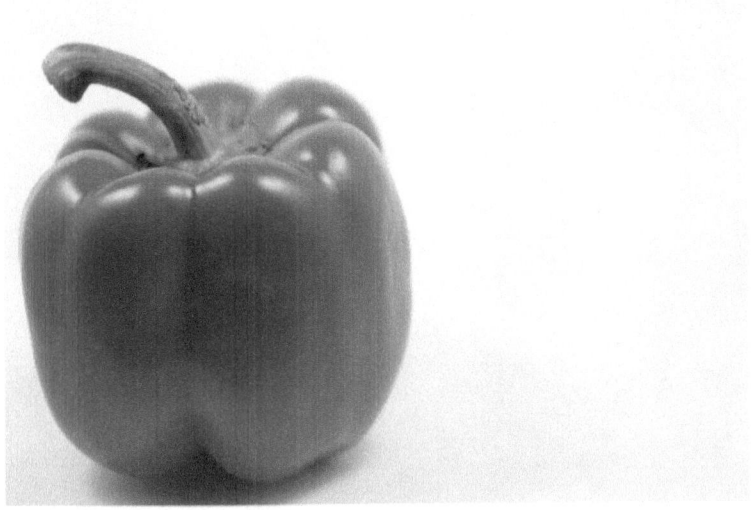

½ cup pepper contains:

- Potassium: only 88 Milligram
- Sodium: only 1 Milligram
- Phosphorus: only 10 Milligram

You can include bell pepper in your diet because it is low in potassium and high in other flavors. Bell peppers are an excellent source of Vitamin A and C, fiber, Vitamin B6 and folic acid. Red Bell peppers are useful for you because they have lycopene to protect your body against particular cancers.

You can mix red pepper in chicken and tuna salad; enjoy as an appetizer or snack or enhance the taste of your omelet by adding chopped red pepper.

(4) Cauliflower

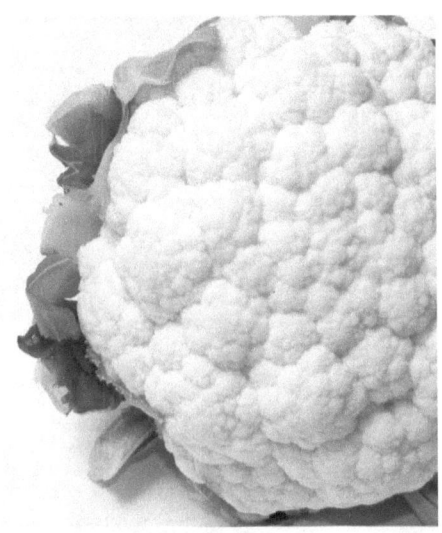

Only ½ cup of cauliflower has 88-milligram potassium, 9-milligram sodium, and 20-milligram phosphorus.

Cauliflower is a great source of fiber, folate, and vitamin C. It is packed with glucosinolates, indoles and thiocyanates. It is good to neutralize the toxicity of liver because the toxic substance can damage DNA and cell membranes.

Enjoy it as a salad with dip or boil or steam cauliflower with curry powder, turmeric, herbal seasoning, and pepper. The nondairy white mush will be a good choice to enjoy pasta with cauliflower and mash cauliflower.

(5) Onions

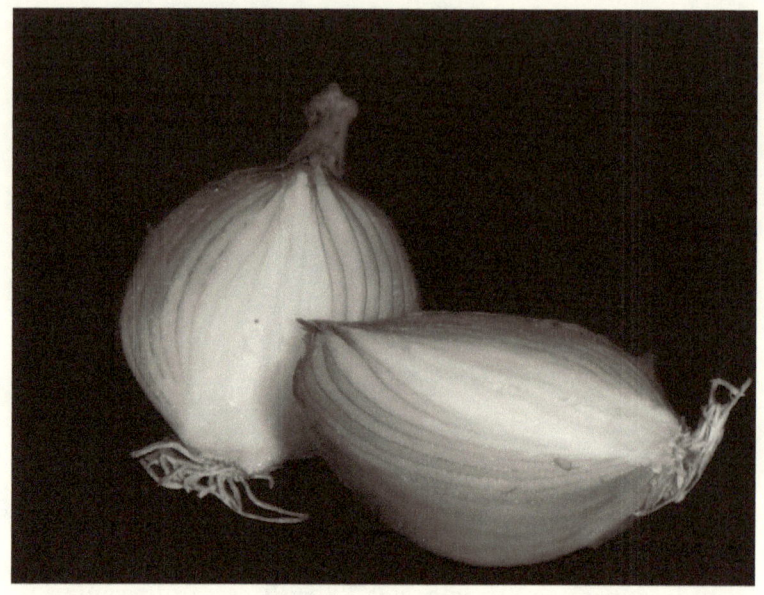

Only ½ cup chopped onion contains 116 milligrams potassium, 3 milligrams phosphorus, and 3 milligrams sodium. Onions are packed with flavonoids and quercetin. This powerful antioxidant can reduce heart diseases and decrease the chances of cancer. These are low in potassium, a good source of mineral and chromium. Onions are helpful to metabolize fat, carbohydrates, and protein.

(6) Apples

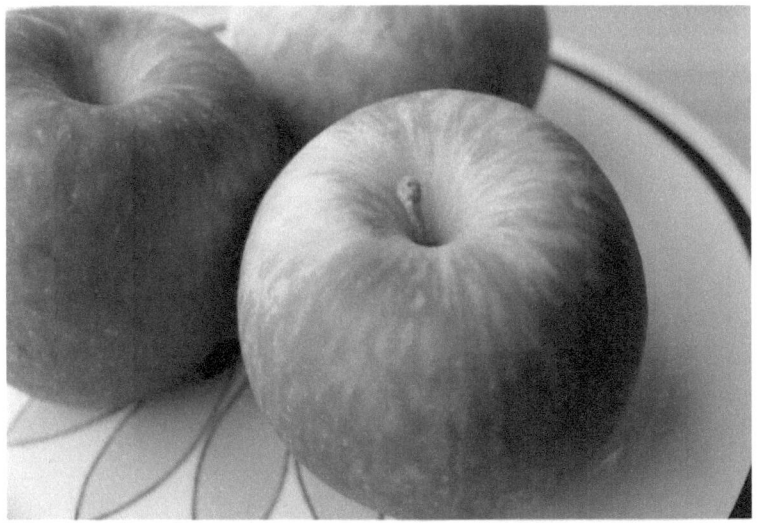

1 apple of medium size with skin contains 10-milligram phosphorus, 0 sodium, and 158 milligrams potassium. It is good to use apples to avoid heart problems, cancer, and constipation and reduce cholesterol.

(7) Cranberries

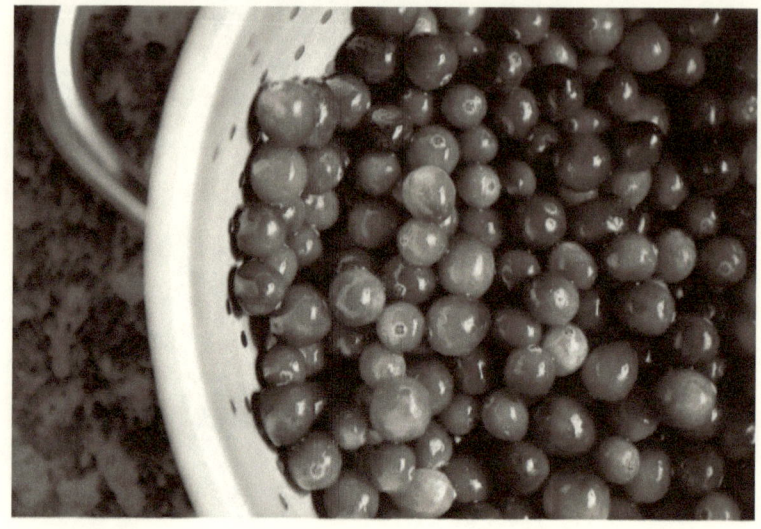

Only ½ cup of dry cranberries has 24 milligrams potassium, 5-milligram phosphorus, and 2 milligrams sodium. In ½ cup cranberry cocktail juice, you will find 3-milligram phosphorus, 22-milligram potassium, and 3 milligrams sodium. Cranberries are useful to protect you from a stomach ulcer, cancer and heart problems.

(8) Strawberries

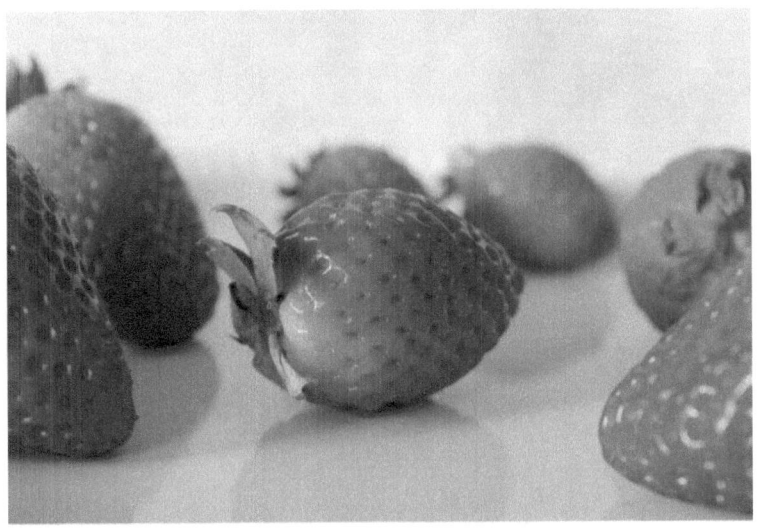

In ½ cup of fresh strawberries, you will get 120 milligrams potassium, 1-milligram sodium, and 13 milligrams phosphorus. The red color indicates that strawberries have powerful antioxidant for the protection of your body structure. These are a good source of vitamin C, fiber, manganese, B vitamin, folate and lots of other nutrients.

Moreover, you can include red grapes, cherries, egg whites, fish, and olive oil because these are low in phosphorus, potassium, and sodium. These food items are good for patients suffering from kidney disease.

(9) Raspberries

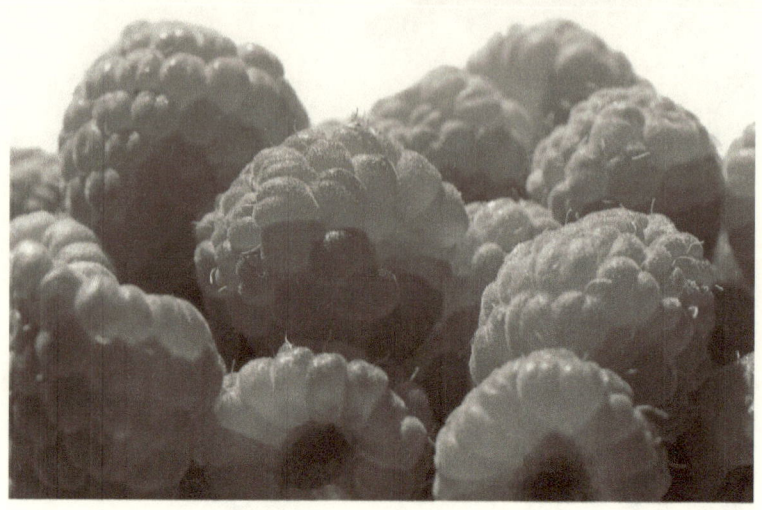

In ½ cup of raspberries, you can find 93 milligrams potassium, 0-milligram sodium, and 7 milligrams phosphorus. These contain ellagic acid to reduce the amount of free radicals in your body and avoid cell damage. These are packed with vitamin C, fiber, manganese, B vitamin, folate and lots of other nutrients.

(10) Blueberries

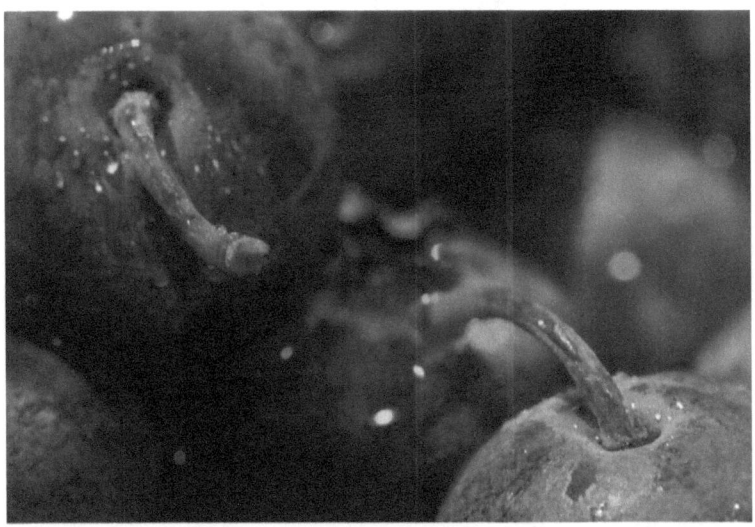

In ½ cup of fresh blueberries, you can find 65 milligrams potassium, 4-milligram sodium, and 7-milligram phosphorus. These berries have anthocyanidins and phytonutrients. These are packed with manganese, vitamin C and fiber. These are good to protect your bones and brain.

Chapter II: Kidney Friendly Breakfast

xxxxxxxxxxxxxxxxxxxxxxxxxxxxxxx

Kidney patients should reduce potassium, phosphorus, and sodium in their diet. There are a few smoothies that can be a good addition to your diet:

Recipe 1: Parsley and Apple for Allergies

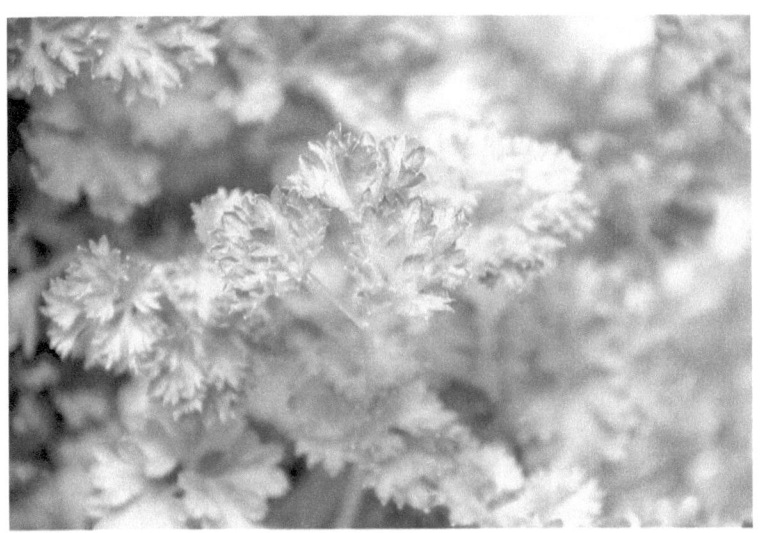

List of Ingredients:

- 2 cups parsley, flat-leaf
- 2 medium lemons, remove peels
- 1 green apple
- 1 ginger knob (optional)

xxxxxxxxxxxxxxxxxxxxxxxxxxxxxxxx

Instructions:

Process all ingredients in your juicer and strain this juice. You can add more apples to enhance its taste. With the help of some filtered water, you can dilute this juice.

Health Benefits: of Parsley

With vitamins A, B, K, C and B 12, parsley can improve your immune system, heal your nervous system, and reduce blood pressure and tone your bones. It is good to detox your body and flush excessive fluid from the body to support kidney function.

Recipe 2: Cucumber and Ginger Juice

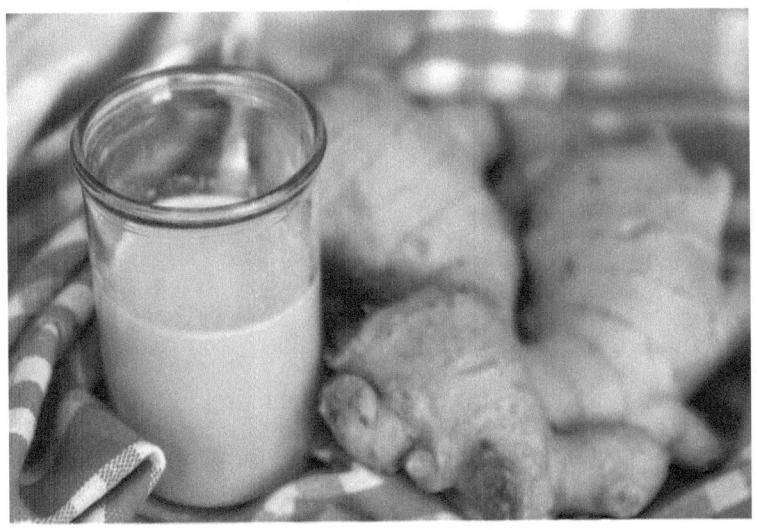

List of Ingredients:

- 1-inch fresh ginger, remove skin and chopped
- 1 cucumber, remove peels and chopped
- Lemon slice, to garnish
- Cucumber slice, to garnish

xxxxxxxxxxxxxxxxxxxxxxxxxxxxxxx

Instructions:

Use a food processor or blender and blend ginger and cucumber together. Now, you can add ½ cup chilled water and strain it using a mesh sieve. You can extract the juice by pressing puree and serve it with ice and lemon juice.

Health Benefits:

Cucumber juice will keep you hydrated, fight with inner heat and helpful to treat heartburn. This juice can be applied on the skin to treat sunburn. A glass of cucumber juice will be helpful to reduce weight. By drinking cucumber juice, you can stabilize blood pressure, cut cancer and refresh your mouth.

Recipe 3: Chocolate Cream Shake with lots of Fibers

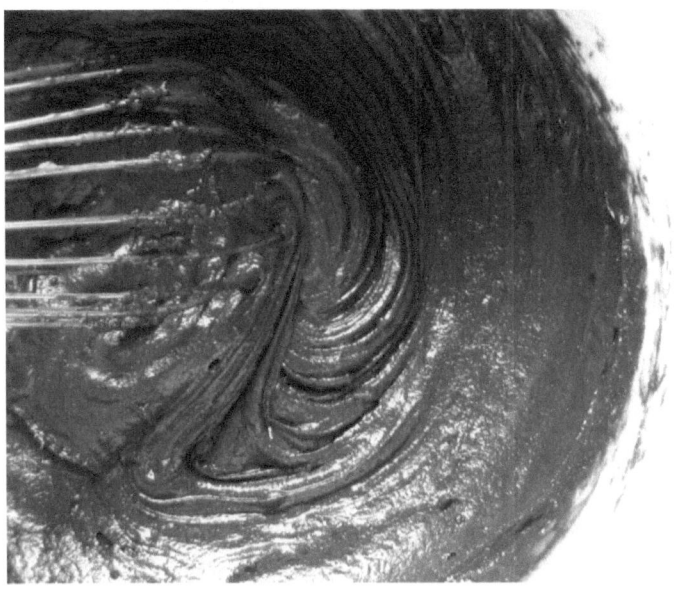

List of Ingredients:

- Protein powder (low carb) 25g
- Cooking cream with 35% fat, 100ml
- Dark cocoa powder without sugar, 1 tsp.
- Sesame oil, 1 Tbsp.
- Psyllium husk, 1 tsp.
- Liquid sweetener, almost 5 to 6 drops

xxxxxxxxxxxxxxxxxxxxxxxxxxxxxxxx

Instructions:

Take 300ml water and properly mix cocoa, psyllium husk and protein powder into it. Now you will add sesame oil and sweetener. Whisk it again and then adds cream. It is time to mix it well, but avoid foaming that can be formed as a result of the shaking. You should drink it within 30 minutes after making it.

Health Benefits:

This will be a good addition in your kidney diet with all healthy ingredients.

Recipe 4: Ginger Detoxification

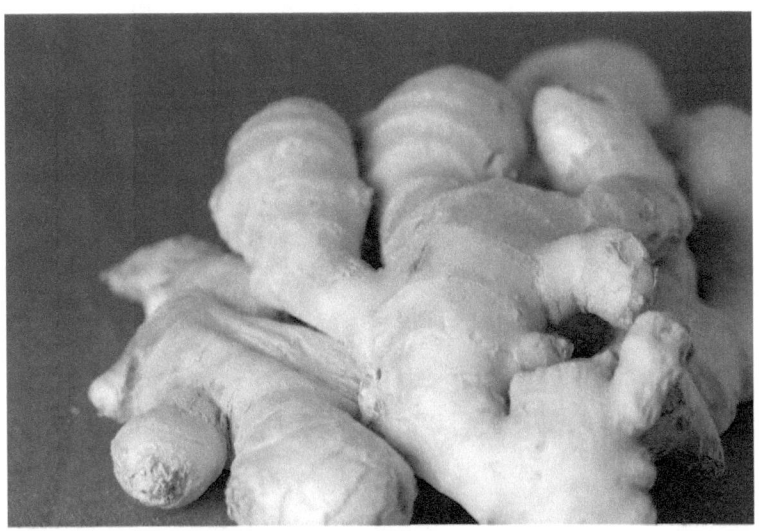

List of Ingredients:

- Cucumber (chopped) – ½ cup
- Baby cabbage – ½ cup
- Minced ginger – 2 Tbsp.
- Lemon Juice - 1 Tbsp.
- Plain yogurt – 1 cup

xxxxxxxxxxxxxxxxxxxxxxxxxxxxxx

Instructions:

Cucumber and ginger will be an amazing combination to reduce weight. It is good to reduce fatigue and sluggishness of your body. Ginger has antibiotics that can be a part of your body. It is really easy to make a blend by putting all the ingredients in a blender. It will be a perfect drink for detoxification.

Health Benefits:

This smoothie is good for the patients suffering from kidney disease because it has all useful ingredients.

Recipe 5: Zucchini and Pear Juice Recipe

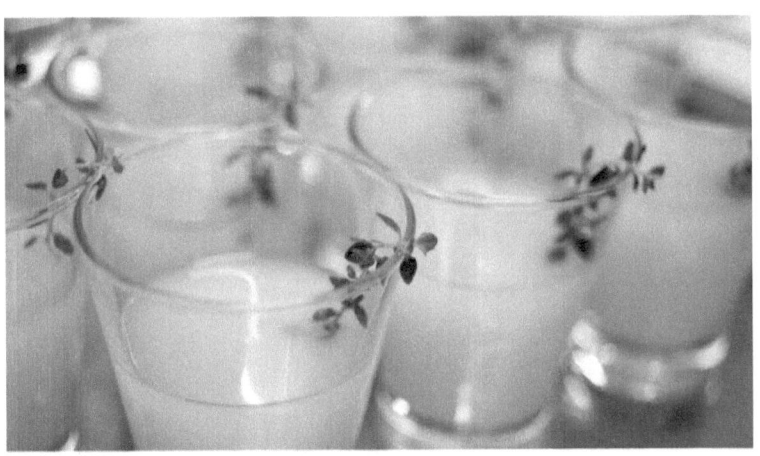

List of Ingredients:

- A handful of dandelion leaves
- 1 lemon
- 1 Zucchini
- 1 Pear
- 1 cucumber

XXXXXXXXXXXXXXXXXXXXXXXXXXXXXX

Instructions:

Wash all ingredients and cut all produce to easily fit through juicer. Pour ice in the juice and enjoy.

Health Benefits:

These are technically famous as a weed and these are famous for their powerful Health Benefits, such as detoxification, normalize blood sugar and relieve allergy.

Recipe 6: Apple and Watercress Juices

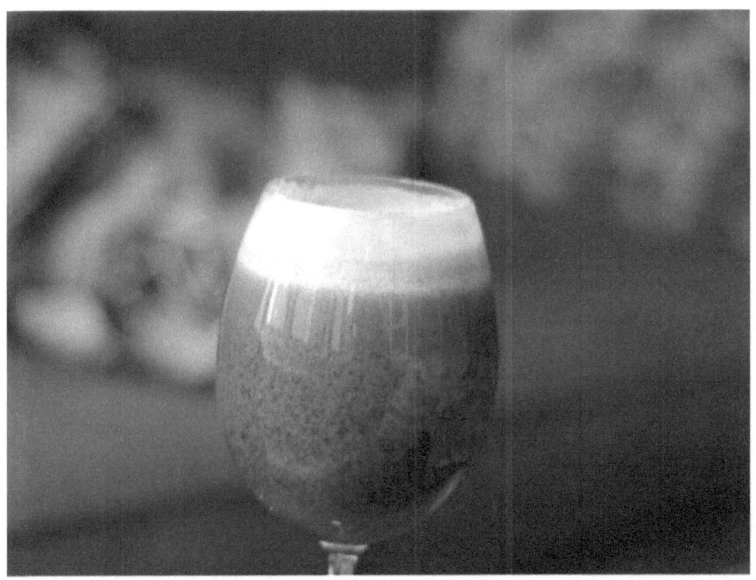

List of Ingredients:

- 1 bunch of watercress
- 1 lime
- 2 green apples
- 2 stalks of celery

xxxxxxxxxxxxxxxxxxxxxxxxxxxxxx

Instructions:

Wash all fruits and vegetables and peel the lime. Process all ingredients through a juicer and enjoy with ice.

Health Benefits:

Green apples are really beneficial for all of you to improve your kidney disease.

Recipe 7: Dandelion and Orange Juice Recipe

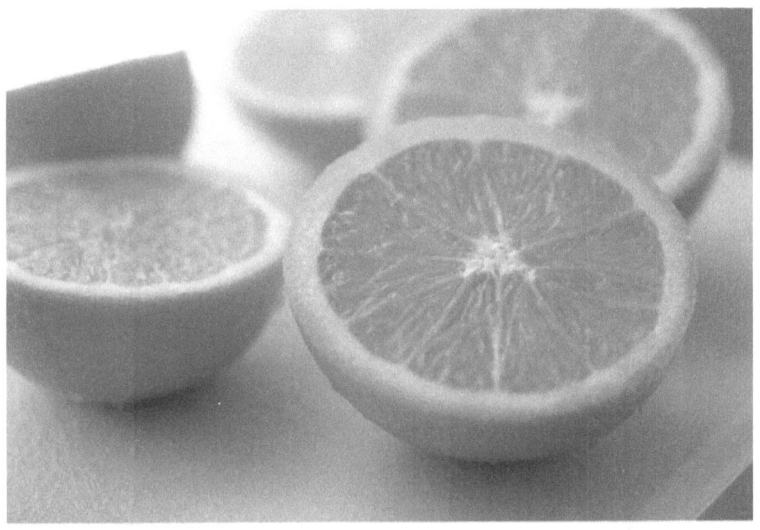

List of Ingredients:

- A handful of dandelion leaves
- 1 lemon
- 2 celery sticks
- 1 cucumber
- 1 Orange (remove skin)

xxxxxxxxxxxxxxxxxxxxxxxxxxxxxx

Instructions:

Wash all ingredients and cut all produce to easily fit through juicer. Pour ice in the juice and enjoy.

Health Benefits:

These are technically famous as a weed and these are famous for their powerful Health Benefits:, such as detoxification, normalize blood sugar and relieve allergy.

Recipe 8: Pear and Parsley Juice

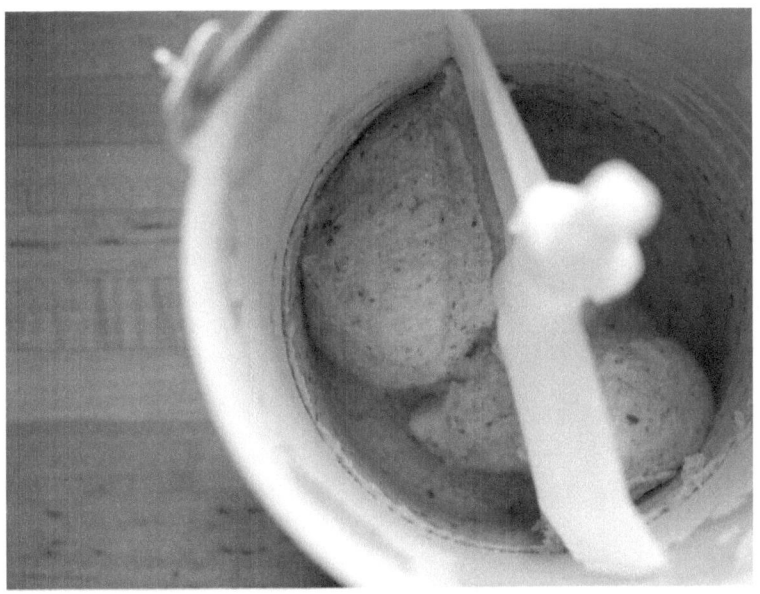

List of Ingredients:

- ½ cup parsley
- ½ lemon, remove rind
- 6 large celery stalks, trimmed
- 2 medium pears, cut
- Ice cubes

xxxxxxxxxxxxxxxxxxxxxxxxxxxxxx

Instructions:

Start with parsley, and then process lemon, pears, cabbage and celery through your juicer. It will be good to follow the directions of the manufacturer. You can fill your glasses with ice before pouring juice and then serve immediately.

Health Benefits:

Parsley is good for the treatment of urinary tract, kidney stones, and other health conditions.

Recipe 9: Turnip and Pear Juice

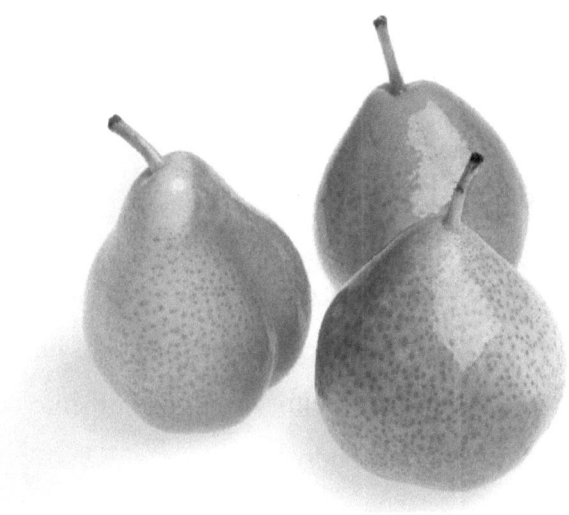

List of Ingredients:

- 1 turnip
- ½ cucumber
- 1 pear
- ¼ cantaloupe, remove skin
- 1 large carrot

xxxxxxxxxxxxxxxxxxxxxxxxxxxxxxx

Instructions:

Wash all ingredients and remove the skin from your cantaloupe. Now, add all ingredients in a juicer to process them. Serve with ice and enjoy.

Health Benefits:

Turnip greens is a great source of vitamin A, K, C and folate, manganese, copper, beta-carotene, vitamin E, B6, fiber and calcium, magnesium, potassium, iron, pantothenic acid, iron, Vitamin B2, and phosphorus.

Recipe 10: Dandelion Juice Recipe with Apple

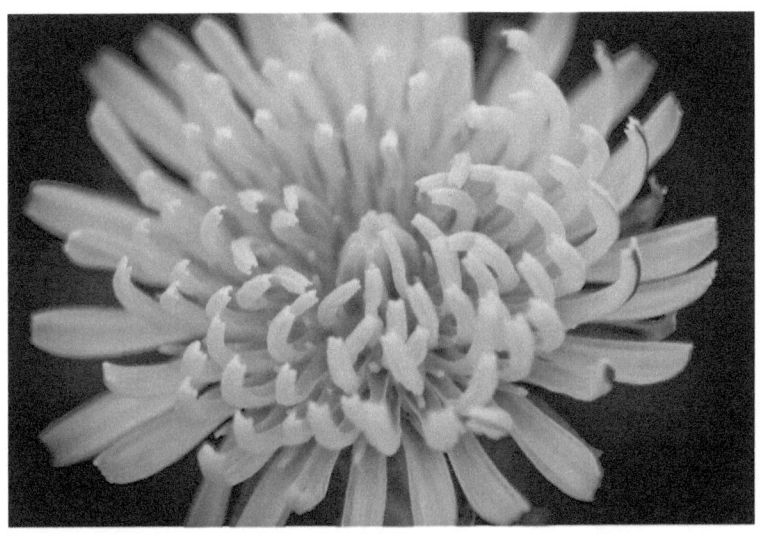

List of Ingredients:

- A handful of dandelion leaves
- 1 lemon
- 2 celery sticks
- 1 cucumber
- 2 green apples

xxxxxxxxxxxxxxxxxxxxxxxxxxxxxxxx

Instructions:

Wash all ingredients and cut all produce to easily fit through juicer. Pour ice in the juice and enjoy.

Health Benefits:

These are technically famous as a weed and these are famous for their powerful Health Benefits:, such as detoxification, normalize blood sugar and relieve allergy.

Chapter III: Kidney Friendly Lunch

xxxxxxxxxxxxxxxxxxxxxxxxxxxxxxx

There are a few recipes for lunches for kidney patients. If you are suffering from kidney diseases, you can get the advantage of these recipes.

Recipe 11: Special Cabbage Soup

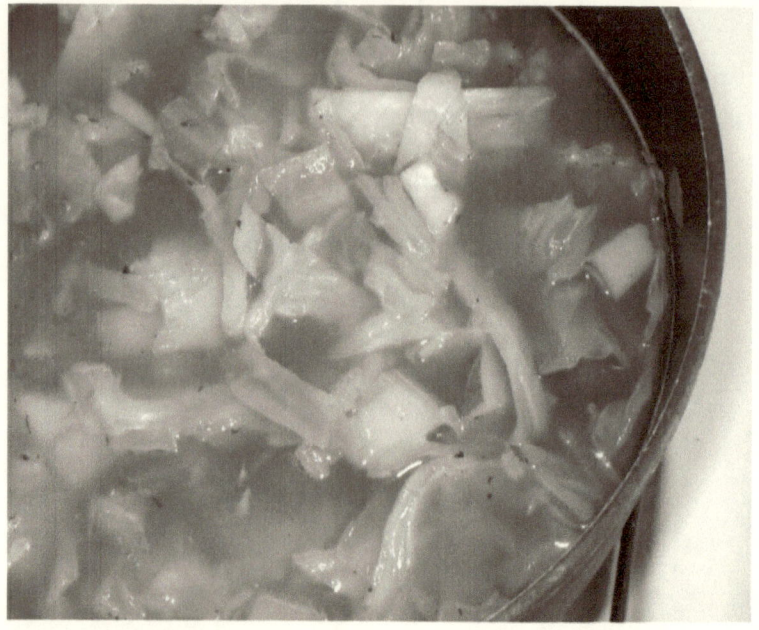

Cooking Time: 45 Minutes

Serving: 4 to 6 People

List of Ingredients:

- 2 garlic cloves, chopped
- 3 cups beef broth (no salt and fat)
- ½ onion
- 2 cups sliced cabbage
- ½ cup beans (green)

- ½ tsp. basil
- ½ cup sliced carrot
- ½ tsp. oregano
- ½ cup sliced zucchini
- Salt and pepper (low)

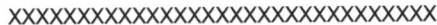

xxxxxxxxxxxxxxxxxxxxxxxxxxxxxxx

Instructions:

Grease a nonstick cooking pot and cook onion, garlic and carrot for 5 minutes. Now cook cabbage, basil, beans, oregano, broth, salt and pepper for almost 10 minutes. The zucchini can be cooked for another 5 minutes to make it tender. You can add or subtract different vegetables as per your taste. You can use green onion instead of yellow onion.

Health Benefits:

Cabbage is really beneficial for people suffering from kidney problems. You can enjoy this soup in lunch or dinner.

Recipe 12: Tuna Sandwiches

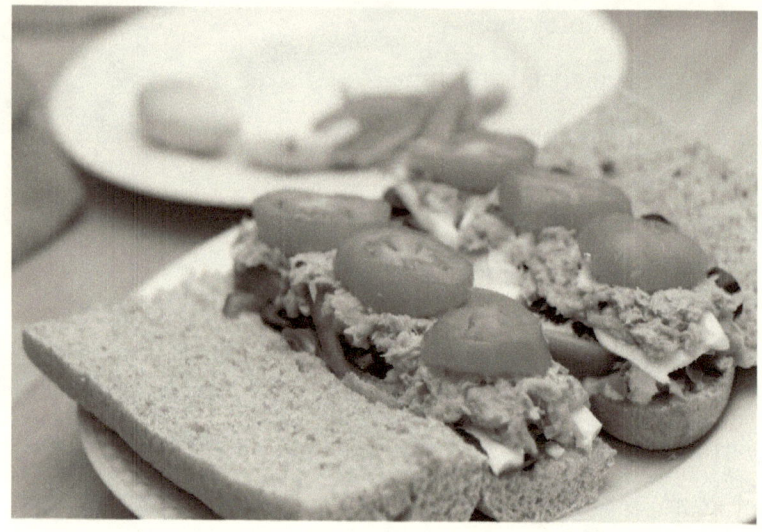

Cooking Time: 10 Minutes

List of Ingredients:

- 6 oz tuna fish, drain liquid
- 2 Tbsp. chopped parsley
- ½ grated carrots, raw
- 2 Tbsp. mayonnaise, low fat, and salt
- 1 Tbsp. lime juice, fresh
- 1 raw shallot, shredded
- 1 tsp. lemon zest
- 4 slices of wheat bread
- ½ cup arugula
- ½ tsp. black pepper

XXXXXXXXXXXXXXXXXXXXXXXXXXXXXXX

Instructions:

Prepare a mixture of all ingredients in a bowl other than bread and arugula. Top 2 slices with ½ cup tuna mixture, ¼ cup arugula, and remaining slices.

Health Benefits:

Tuna is good for kidney patients and this recipe will be really good for your health.

Recipe 13: Brewery Burger

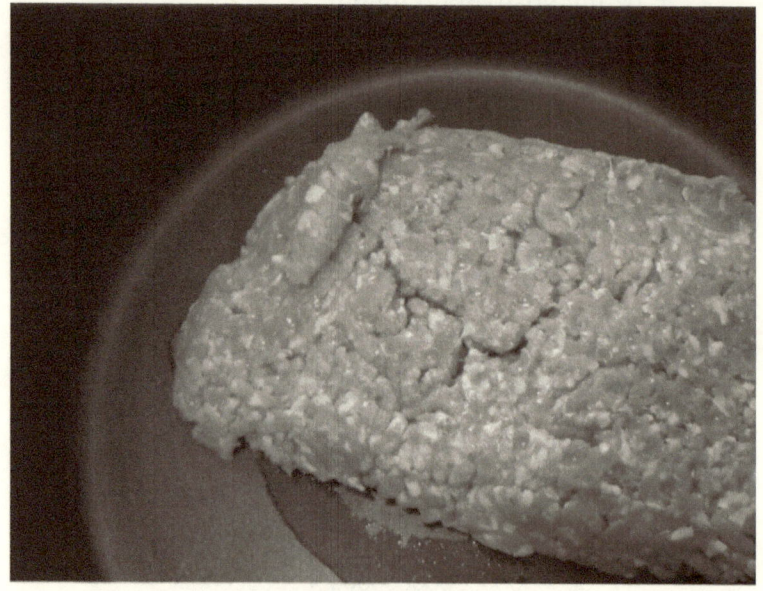

Serving Size: 3 ½ ounces (cooked)

Cooking Time:0 Depends on You

Ingredients

- Rice Milk: 3 Tbsp.
- Egg: 1
- 5 crackers: free from salt and soda
- Herbal seasoning mixture: 1 tsp.
- Ground beef: 1 pound

XXXXXXXXXXXXXXXXXXXXXXXXXXXXXX

Instructions:

Prepare a mixture of crushed crackers and milk in a bowl and leave it for some time. Meanwhile, beat eggs and add herbal blend, eggs, and beef in the mixture of crackers. It is time to divide it to make four equal sizes of patties and grill it on the medium flame until you cook it to your desired level.

Health Benefits:

These burgers are healthy for a patient suffering from kidney diseases. You should try them.

Recipe 14: Barbecued Joes

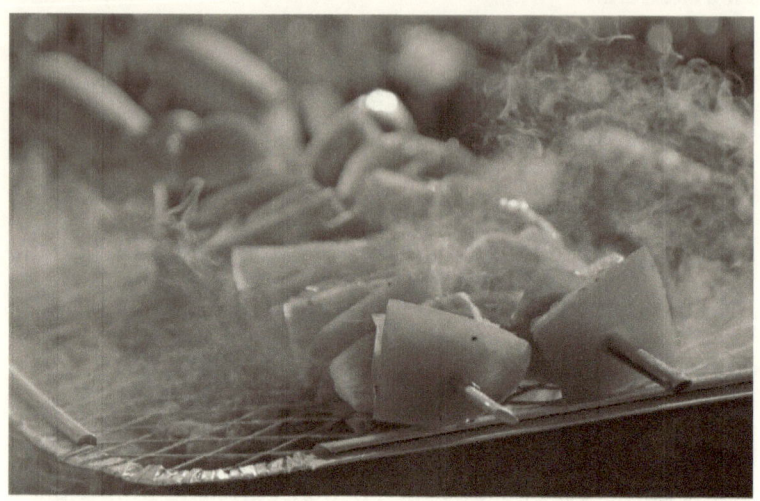

Cooking Time: 30 Minute

List of Ingredients:

- 1 pound raw turkey breast
- ½ tsp. cayenne pepper
- ½ chopped bell pepper
- ½ chopped onion
- ½ chopped red pepper
- 1 cup barbecue sauce
- 4-grain hamburger rolls, sliced

xxxxxxxxxxxxxxxxxxxxxxxxxxxxxxxx

Instructions:

Great a nonstick cooking pan with cooking oil and add the turkey to let it brown. It may take almost 10 minutes. Remove any liquid and add onion and peppers to cook almost 3 minutes. Add cayenne pepper and barbecue sauces and cook for almost 2 minutes. Take one-half of the half and top with turkey mixture and cover with another half of the bun. Serve with a low fat and low sugar sauce.

Health Benefits:

Bell pepper and onion are really good for your health and improve your kidney disease.

Recipe 15: Lemon Chicken and Broccoli

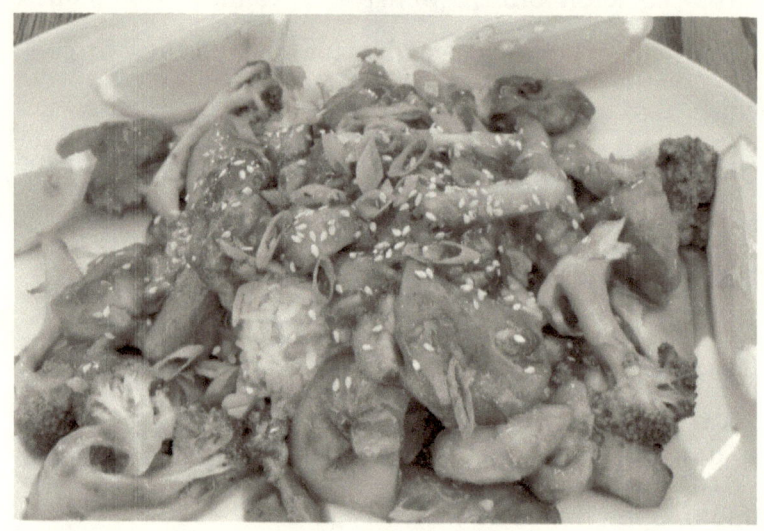

Cooking Time: 1 Hour

Serving: 4

Ingredients

- 2 Tbsp. flour (all-purpose)
- 1/4 tsp. black pepper powder
- 12 oz chicken breast(s), chopped
- ½ tsp. table salt, (divided)
- 2 tsp. olive oil
- 2 ½ cups raw broccoli, take small floret
- 2 tsp. garlic paste
- 1 ½ cups chicken broth, (divided, without salt and fat)
- 2 tsp. lemon zest as per taste
- 1 Tbsp. lemon juice
- 2 Tbsp. chopped parsley

xxxxxxxxxxxxxxxxxxxxxxxxxxxxxx

Instructions:

Mix 1.5 Tbsp. flour, salt and pepper (1/4 tsp.) and chicken in a bowl.

Take a nonstick pan and pour oil to keep it on a medium heat. It is time to add chicken and cook for five minutes to make it light brown. Now remove it in the plate.

Now cook 1 cup broth along with garlic paste in the pan. Let it boil on a high heat and use a wooden spoon to scrape the brown bits from the bottom. Now add the broccoli and cook for one minute.

Take a small cup and mix ½ Tbsp. flour, remaining broth and ¼ tsp. salt. Now add to the skillet and let it cook on the low heat. Cover it and cook to make a thick sauce and let the broccoli soft. It will take almost 1.5minutes. Mix chicken and lemon zest while heating.

Remove pan from the heat and mix parsley and lime juice; mix well. Its serving size is one cup.

Health Benefits:

All ingredients in this recipe are friendly for kidney patients and gradually improve your health.

Recipe 16: Chicken Sandwich

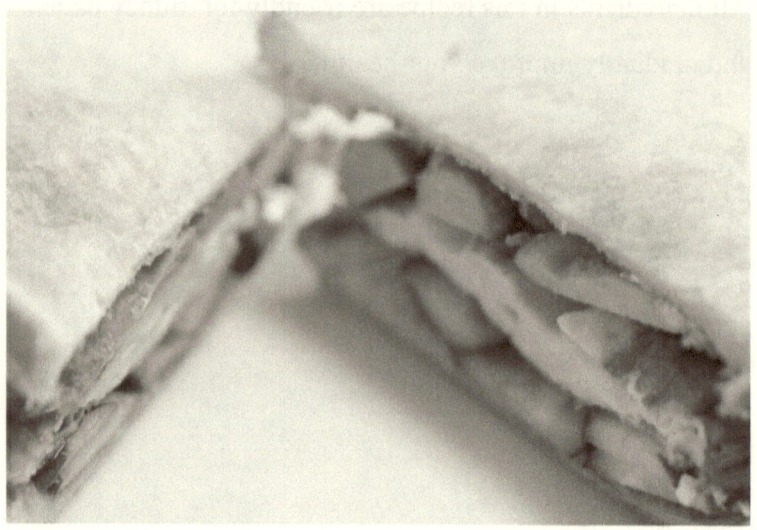

Cooking Time: 40 to 50 minutes

Serving Size: 2 Servings

List of Ingredients:

- ¼ cup fat-free salad dressing
- 1/3 cup bread crumbs
- 1-pound boneless chicken breast
- ¼ cup shredded cheese
- ½ cup vegetable sauce
- 8 slices of bread, low calorie

XXXXXXXXXXXXXXXXXXXXXXXXXXXXXXX

Instructions:

Prepare one in advance at 400°F. Meanwhile, grease a baking pan with cooking oil. Keep Italian dressing and crumbs in deep bowls. Coat chicken with dressing and bread crumbs, one by one. Keep the chicken in greased pan and bake for 15 minutes. Place chili sauce and cheese on the top and bake it for another 10 minutes. Keep the each slice of chicken in bread and top it with another bread before serving. You can use low fat and low sugar sauce to enjoy sandwiches.

Health Benefits:

These sandwiches are really healthy for you because it is free from any harmful ingredient. This will be a good addition in your diet.

Recipe 17: Tortellini Soup in Crock Pot

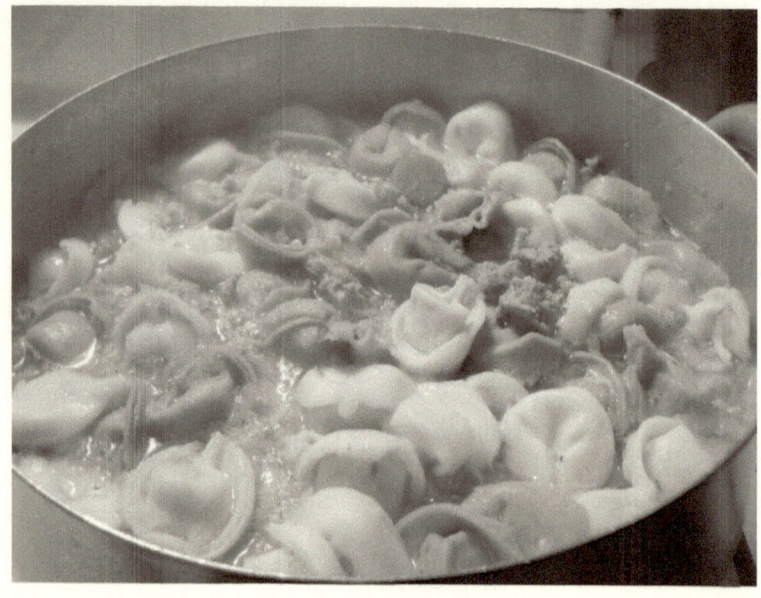

Cooking Time: 3 to 4 hours in crock pot on low setting

Serving Size: 4 people

Ingredients

- 3 cups broth (chicken)
- 1 cup water
- 8-10 oz. Tortellini pasta
- 1 chopped onion, small
- 1 tsp. Basil
- 2 fresh stalks of celery
- ¼ cup cheese
- 3 cloves crushed garlic
- 1 tsp. pepper (black)
- 1 tsp. Basil
- 1½ cups chopped cabbage
- 1 tsp. Oregano
- 1 tsp. Rosemary
- 1 Tbsp. olive oil

XXXXXXXXXXXXXXXXXXXXXXXXXXXXXX

Instructions:

Take a pan and pour olive oil to cook celery, onions, and carrots on a medium heat to make onions soft. Mix garlic in these ingredients and cook for 2 to 3 minutes. Now add tomatoes, water, rosemary, broth, oregano and black pepper to cook for five minutes.

It is time to add cabbage, cheese and pasta to cook for almost 15 minutes and stir several times while cooking.

Instructions to Cook in Crock Pot:

Add garlic, organic, carrot, black pepper, rosemary, water, onions, broth and oregano into crock pot. Cook it on a low setting for 3 to 4 hours. After cooking this, add cabbage, pasta, and cheese to cook for another one hour.

Health Benefits:

These are good to improve your health and prevent lots of health problems from your diet.

Chapter IV: Kidney Friendly Dinner

xxxxxxxxxxxxxxxxxxxxxxxxxxxxxx

In order to make your dinner special, there are a few recipes that are friendly for kidney patients:

Recipe 18: Cod Fillets

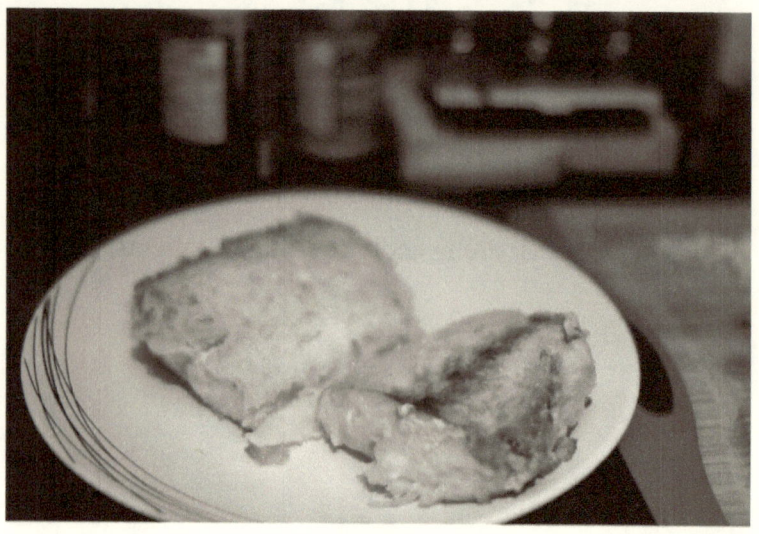

Cooking Time: 2 hours for preparation

15 to 20 minutes for cooking

List of Ingredients:

- 2 raw scallions, crushed
- 1 Tbsp. ginger paste
- 2 tsp. garlic paste
- 1 Tbsp. sherry cooking wine (non-alcoholic)
- 1 Tbsp. soy sauce
- 1.5 pounds raw Pacific cod

XXXXXXXXXXXXXXXXXXXXXXXXXXXXXXX

Instructions:

Keep the fish in a baking dish. Take a small bowl and mix ginger, scallions, garlic, sherry and soy sauce to pour over the fish. Let it marinate for almost 2 hours.

Take a saucepan and fill it with water to keep on a high heat. Let it boil and keep fish in a steamer basket. Now discard marinade and keep the steamer basket in the saucepan. The basket should sit above water.

Steam fish after covering the saucepan and wait for its complete cooking. It should be easy to flake with a fork. It will take almost 10 minutes. Divide into pieces and enjoy.

Health Benefits:

Ginger and pacific code is a good combination for kidney patients

Recipe 19: Baked Red Pepper

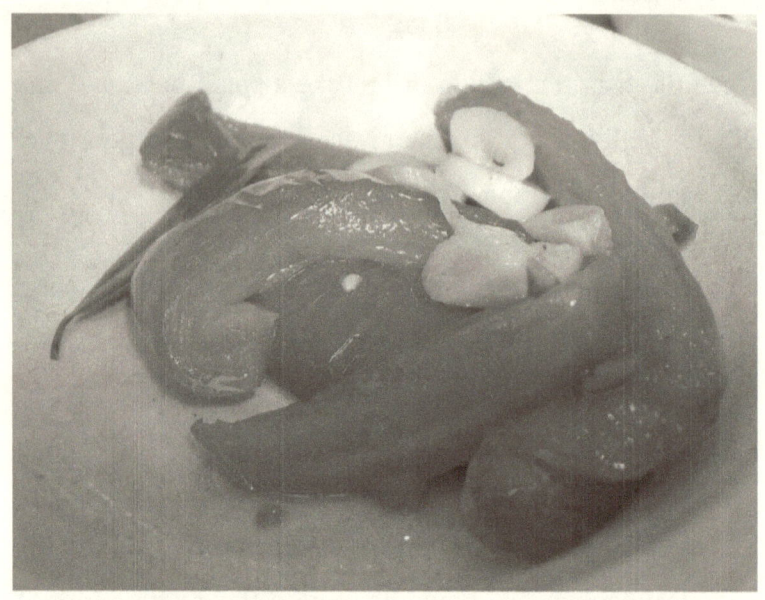

Cooking Time: One Hour

List of Ingredients:

- 4 Red Bell Peppers
- 3 Tbsp. bread crumbs, Italian seasoned
- 3 Tbsp. grated cheese

xxxxxxxxxxxxxxxxxxxxxxxxxxxxxx

Instructions:

Preheat your oven to 350 degrees F or 175 C. Grease a nonstick cooking pan and set aside.

Slice bell peppers in half and removes its seeds and inner material. Now keep these slices in the prepared baking pan. Prepare a mixture of cheese and breadcrumbs in a bowl. Sprinkle this mixture evenly on peppers. Bake it for 35 to 45 minutes to make the topping brown. Serve with your favorite healthy sauce.

Health Benefits:

You can enjoy tasty red bell peppers at dinner without any tension because it is healthy for kidney patients.

Recipe 20: Chicken with Jalapeno Pepper

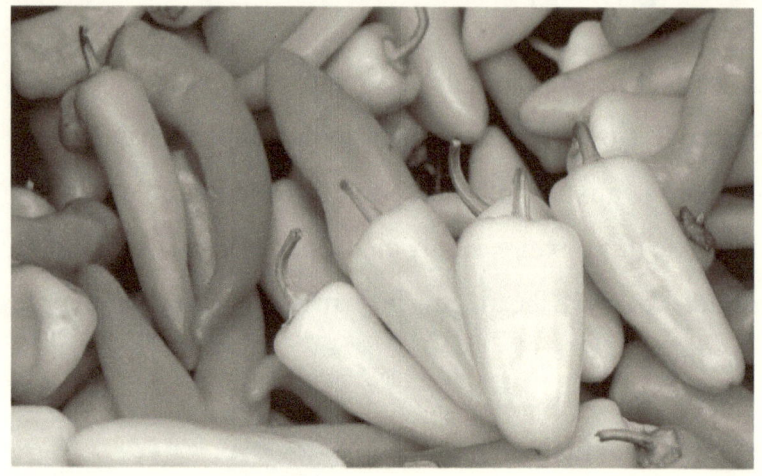

Serving Size: 3-ounces

Total Yield: 8 Servings

List of Ingredients:

- 3 Tbsp. healthy vegetable oil
- 1 onion, sliced
- 2 to 3 pounds skinless chicken, pieces
- 1 ½ cup chicken bouillon without salt
- ¼ tsp. powder of black pepper
- ½ tsp. nutmeg powder
- 2 tsp. chopped jalapeno peppers

XXXXXXXXXXXXXXXXXXXXXXXXXXXXXXX

Instructions:

Let the oil hot in a cooking pan and fry the pieces of chicken to make them brown. Keep them aside in a bowl. Cook onion rings in the oil and adds bouillon to let it boil. Mix it frequently and return the chicken to the pan. Add black pepper and nutmeg, now cover it with a lid and let it simmer for almost 35 minutes. Make sure that the chicken is completely tender. Mix jalapeno peppers and cook it for one minute.

Health Benefits:

It has only 45 mg sodium, 127 mg phosphorus, and 160 mg potassium. It is healthy for you to enjoy with kidney disease.

Recipe 21: Chinese Soup

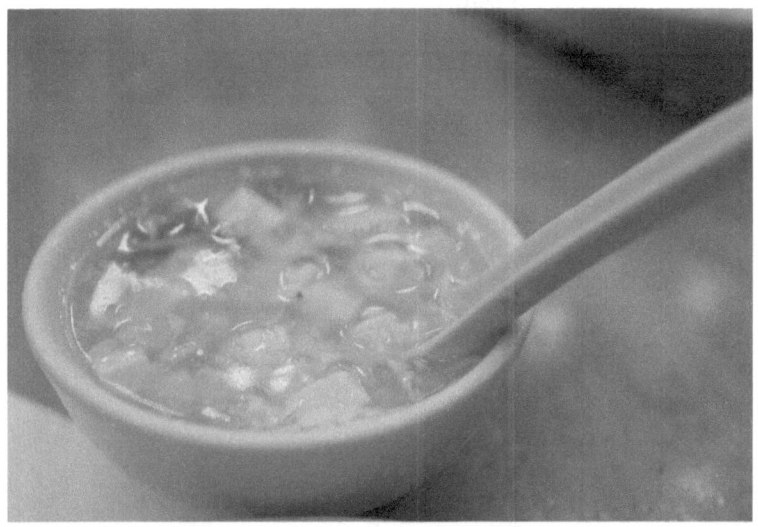

Cooking Time: One hour

Ingredients

- 14 oz coconut milk, light
- 5 cups chicken broth, fat-free
- 1 Tbsp. ginger, crushed
- 4 Tbsp. fish sauce
- 1/4 cup lemongrass, chopped
- 2 Tbsp. sauce (Siracha)
- Two limes, juice
- 2 Tbsp. sugar
- 1/4 cup chopped scallions
- 1 cup peas, (sugar snap)
- 1/4 cup chopped cilantro
- ½ cup broccoli florets
- 2 zucchini, diced
- 1/3 cup carrots, sliced
- 1 cup mushrooms, chopped

xxxxxxxxxxxxxxxxxxxxxxxxxxxxxxx

Instructions:

Take a large pot and add lemon grass, ginger and stock to let it boil. Keep it on a medium heat and cook for 30 minutes. Wait for lemongrass to release yummy flavors. Now add the lime juice, milk, both sauces, and sugar. Cook it for almost 10 minutes.

Meanwhile, blanch zucchini, broccoli and carrots in boiling water for almost 2 minutes. You have to make them a bit soft. Now take 6 bowls and equally divide vegetables. Distribute soups equally into each bowl with the vegetables. Serve with cilantro as a topping.

Health Benefits:

This food is really healthy for kidney patients for the prevention of disease.

Recipe 22: Green Chicken

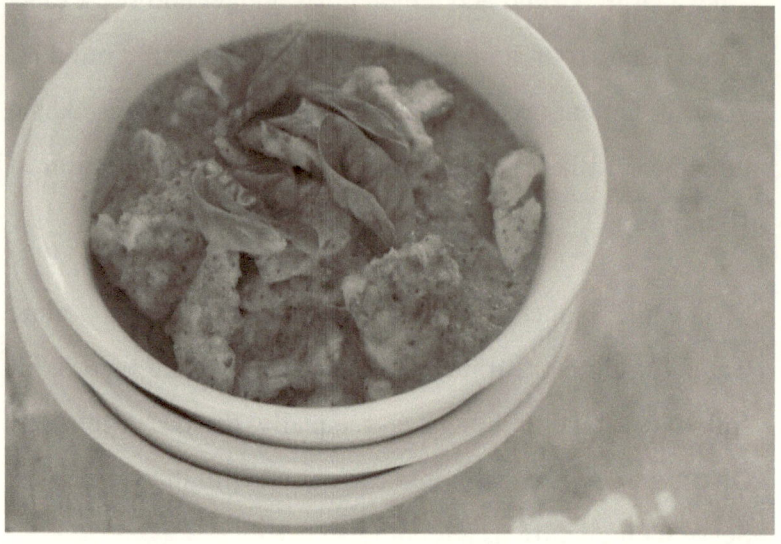

Cooking Time: 4 to 5 Hours

Servings: 2 cups make one serving

List of Ingredients:

- 1 yellow onion, chopped
- 1lb chicken breasts, sliced
- 16oz vegetables of your choice
- 5 garlic cloves, crushed
- 15oz coconut milk, light
- Lemon juice, 1 lime
- 2 Tbsp. brown sugar
- 3 Tbsp. green curry paste
- 1 Tbsp. cornstarch
- ½ tsp. black pepper powder
- 1 tsp. salt

xxxxxxxxxxxxxxxxxxxxxxxxxxxxxx

Instructions:

Put chicken, salt, and pepper in the crock pot and cover it with slices of onion. Take a medium bowl and mix lime juice, coconut milk, sugar, curry paste and add in chicken in the crock pot.

It will take 4 to 5 hours to cook. You can add vegetables in the last 45 minutes of cooking. Take a small bowl to mix cornstarch and 1 Tbsp. of water. Add it to the crock pot along with vegetables and let it heat to make curry sauce thick. One serving is 2 cups.

Health Benefits:

This chicken will be a yummy and healthy addition to your diet to improve your health.

Recipe 23: Grilled Chicken

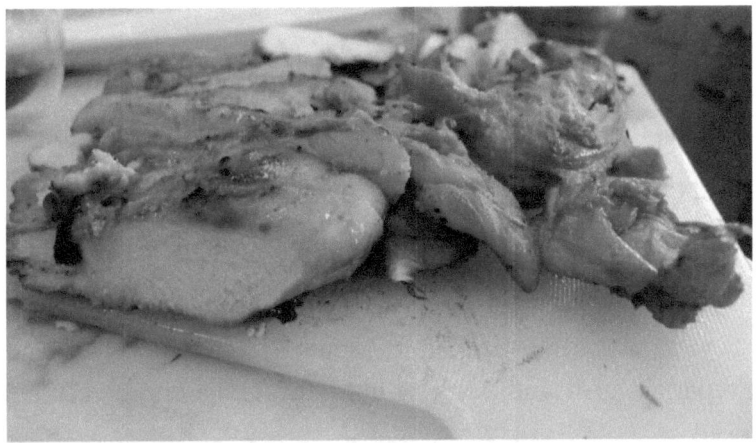

Cooking Time: 3 Hours for Marination and rest of the time in grilling and baking

List of Ingredients:

- 1.5 lbs chicken breasts, 6 fillets (no skin and bone)
- 1 Tbsp. sesame oil
- 1 cup cilantro
- 2 Tbsp. soy sauce, low sodium
- Juice from 1 lime
- 6 garlic cloves
- ½ cup chicken broth, fat-free
- 1 tsp. salt
- ½ tsp. black pepper powder

XXXXXXXXXXXXXXXXXXXXXXXXXXXXXXXX

Instructions:

Process all ingredients except chicken in the food processor to make them smooth. Now keep the chicken in a large bowl and pour blended mixture over the chicken. It should cover all the chicken and now keep it in the refrigerator for almost 3 hours.

Prepare a grill and cook it until the temperature reaches 165F, use a meat thermometer. Keep the breasts on the grill for 5 minutes before enjoying it. Your one serving size will be one chicken breast.

Health Benefits:

Healthy ingredients of this recipe make it really special for all kidney patients.

Recipe 24: Fried Chicken in Oven

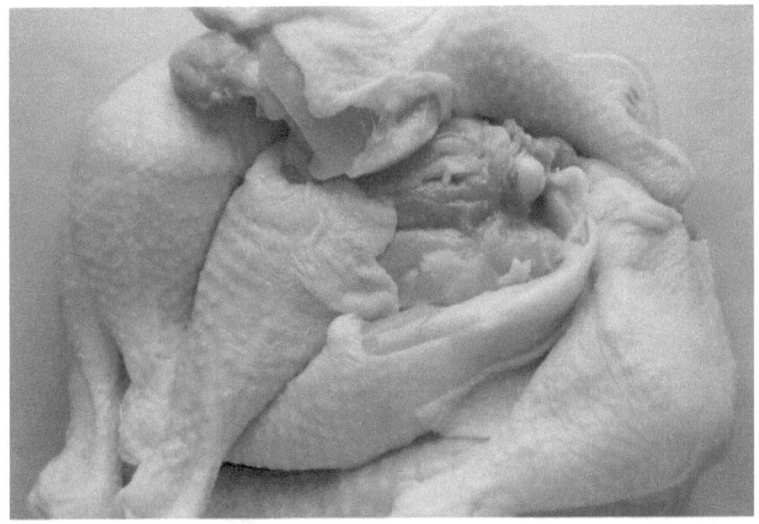

Serving Size: 3 to 4 Ounce

Yield: 8 Pieces

List of Ingredients:

- 1 Tbsp. powder of black pepper
- 2 ½ pound chicken (without skin and fat)
- All-purpose-flour: 1 cup
- Chopped corn flakes: 1 cup
- Vegetable oil: 4 Tbsp.
- Lemon juice: 1 Tbsp.
- Black pepper powder: 1 tsp.
- Poultry seasoning: ¼ tsp.

XXXXXXXXXXXXXXXXXXXXXXXXXXXXXXX

Instructions:

Heat an oven in advance at 400°F. You have to wash the chicken and pat it to dry all moisture. Rub lemon juice all over your chicken. Take a small bag and add black pepper, flour, corn flakes, seasoning and shake it well.

Take a shallow pan for baking that should be 1 inches deep. Grease this pan with your vegetable oil. Add chicken in the bag of dry ingredients and shake well. Carefully arrange all coated pieces in the pan and let them brown for 20 to 30 minutes. You can enjoy with your favorite sauce, but avoid tomato sauce.

Health Benefits:

There is no harm in trying this recipe with kidney problem because it is safe and healthy for everyone.

About the Author

Heston Brown is an accomplished chef and successful e-book author from Palo Alto California. After studying cooking at The New England Culinary Institute, Heston stopped briefly in Chicago where he was offered head chef at some of the city's most prestigious restaurants. Brown decide that he missed the rolling hills and sunny weather of California and moved back to his home state to open up his own catering company and give private cooking classes.

Heston lives in California with his beautiful wife of 18 years and his two daughters who also have aspirations to follow in their father's footsteps and pursue careers in the culinary arts. Brown is well known for his delicious fish and chicken dishes and teaches these recipes as well as many others to his students.

When Heston gave up his successful chef position in Chicago and moved back to California, a friend suggested he use the internet to share his recipes with the world and so he did! To date, Heston Brown has written over 1000 e-books that contain recipes, cooking tips, business strategies for catering companies and a self-help book he wrote from personal experience.

He claims his wife has been his inspiration throughout many of his endeavours and continues to be his partner in business as well as life. His greatest joy is having all three women in his life in the kitchen with him cooking their favourite meal while his favourite jazz music plays in the background.

Author's Afterthoughts

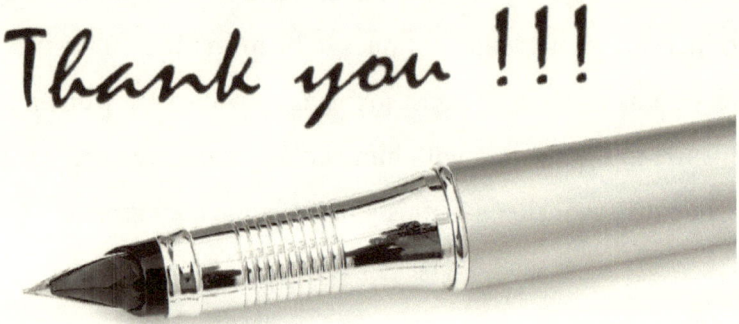

Thank you to all the readers who invested time and money into my book! I cherish every one of you and hope you took the same pleasure in reading it as I did in writing it.

Out of all of the books out there, you chose mine and for that I am truly grateful. It makes the effort worth it when I know my readers are enjoying my work from beginning to end.

Please take a few minutes to write an Amazon review so that others can benefit from your opinions and insight. Your review will help countless other readers make an informed choice

Thank you so much,

Heston Brown

www.ingramcontent.com/pod-product-compliance
Lightning Source LLC
Chambersburg PA
CBHW021237280526
45784CB00005B/2122